# BIOHAZARD BREAKDOWN

## BATTLING BIOLOGICAL BLIGHTS

### Specialist Remediation Solutions Ltd

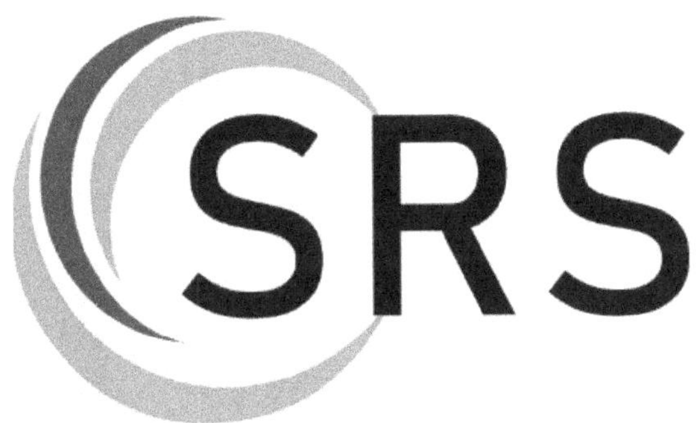

# Contents

# ABOUT THIS BOOK

Biohazard remediation is a critical field that deals with the cleaning, sanitising, and restoring of areas where biological hazards, such as infectious diseases, blood, and other bodily fluids, are present. The importance of this work cannot be overstated, as it directly impacts public health, safety, and environmental integrity. In the United Kingdom, this field is governed by stringent regulations and standards, necessitating a high level of expertise and professionalism.

This book is designed to provide an in-depth understanding of biohazard remediation, specifically tailored to the needs and concerns of commercial clients and dutyholder's. We will explore the various types of biohazards, including crime scene residues, trauma scenes, unattended deaths, and more. Our goal is to provide a comprehensive guide that not only details the technical aspects of remediation but also sheds light on the legal and ethical considerations involved.

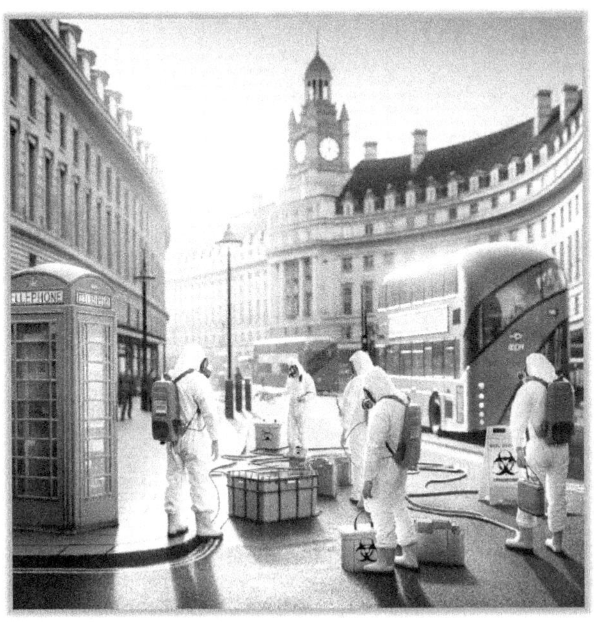

For commercial clients and dutyholder's, the stakes in biohazard remediation are high. Whether it's ensuring a safe working environment, complying with health and safety regulations, or managing the risks associated with biohazard exposure, the responsibilities are significant. This book aims to serve as a valuable resource for understanding these responsibilities and the critical role of choosing the right remediation company.

We will delve into the UK's legal framework governing biohazard remediation, emphasising the dutyholder's obligations and the repercussions of non-compliance. Additionally, we will discuss the importance of qualified and experienced remediation professionals who can ensure safety, efficacy, and compliance with all relevant standards and practices.

In the following chapters, readers will gain insights into the complexities of biohazard remediation. From the initial assessment and planning stages through to the final restoration and post-cleanup validation, every step will be thoroughly examined. Case studies and real-world examples will offer practical insights, and emerging trends and innovations in the field will be explored to keep readers abreast of the latest developments.

This book is more than just a technical guide; it's a comprehensive resource for understanding the critical nature of biohazard remediation and its impact on health, safety, and the environment. It's an essential read for anyone involved in or affected by biohazard cleaning and remediation in the UK.

**Section 1: Understanding Biohazards**

This chapter introduces the concept of biohazards, including their definition, types, and the health and environmental risks they pose. It sets the foundation for understanding the significance of biohazard remediation.

**Section 2: Legal Framework and Compliance**

Focuses on the UK regulations and laws governing biohazard remediation. It details the responsibilities and compliance requirements for dutyholder's, and the consequences of failing to adhere to these regulations.

**Section 3: Biohazard Remediation Process**

Describes the step-by-step process of biohazard remediation, from initial assessment and planning to containment, decontamination, and waste management. It emphasises safe and effective cleanup procedures.

**Section 4: Specific Types of Biohazard Cleaning**

Delves into various specific biohazard scenarios like crime scenes, trauma incidents, and infectious disease outbreaks. It explains the unique challenges and protocols for each type of cleaning situation.

**Section 5: Choosing the Right Remediation Company**

Guides readers on how to select a competent and reliable remediation company. It covers staff qualifications, equipment standards, certifications, and the importance of experience and track record.

**Section 6: Best Practices in Biohazard Remediation**

Discusses the best practices in biohazard remediation, focusing on safety, ethical considerations, quality assurance, and ongoing training and improvement in the field.

## Section 7: Aftermath and Restoration

Covers the steps following the cleanup, including validation of the cleaning process, property restoration, and support resources for psychological impacts.

## Section 8: Case Studies and Real-World Examples

Provides real-world examples and case studies of successful biohazard remediation projects. It includes expert interviews and insights to give readers practical perspectives.

## Section 9: Future Trends and Innovations

Explores emerging technologies, legislative updates, and evolving best practices in biohazard remediation. It gives readers a glimpse into the future of the field.

## Section 10: Resources and Support

Lists additional resources for further reading and education, including government and industry contacts, professional associations, and educational materials.

## Section 11: Global Perspectives and International Cooperation

Emphasises the necessity of global collaboration in managing biohazard incidents, highlighting the role of international organisations, shared resources, and the development of unified standards for effective worldwide biohazard response and remediation.

# ABOUT SRS

We are a trusted provider of high-quality environmental remediation and cleaning services. Our company is based in Desborough, Northamptonshire, and we are proud to serve both residential and commercial clients, nationally across the UK.

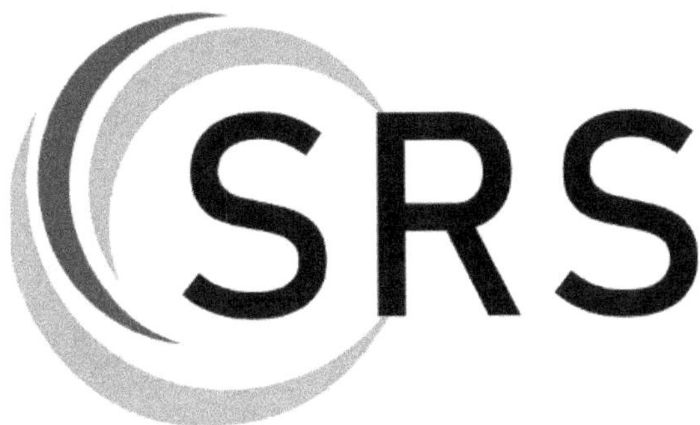

At Specialist Remediation Solutions Ltd, we specialise in four key services: non-licensed and licensed asbestos removal, biohazard cleaning, house clearance, and commercial cleaning.

Our team of experts has the knowledge, skills, and experience to handle even the most challenging environmental remediation and cleaning projects, ensuring that our clients receive the best possible service every time.

We understand that dealing with environmental hazards and cleaning needs can be stressful and overwhelming, which is why we strive to make the process as easy and stress-free as possible. Our team will work closely with you to understand your needs and develop a customised solution that meets your specific requirements. We use only the best equipment, materials, and techniques to ensure that our services are efficient, effective, and safe for all involved. We believe that every client deserves the highest level of service and attention to detail, and we go above and beyond to deliver just that, whatever you need we are here to help.

# UNDERSTANDING BIOHAZARDS

Biohazards, or biological hazards, encompass a broad spectrum of organic materials and agents that pose significant risks to human health and environmental safety. These hazards can originate from a variety of sources, including medical facilities, laboratories, natural occurrences, and human or animal waste. The potential for biohazards to cause illness, environmental damage, and even death underscores the imperative for a thorough understanding and strategic approach to their management and remediation.

## Deep Dive into Common Biohazards in the UK

The UK, with its dense population centres, advanced healthcare system, and diverse ecosystems, encounters a range of biohazard scenarios:

1. **Medical Waste:** The healthcare sector generates sharps, contaminated disposables, and other items that, if mishandled, can spread infections. Effective waste management protocols and strict regulatory compliance are essential to mitigate these risks.

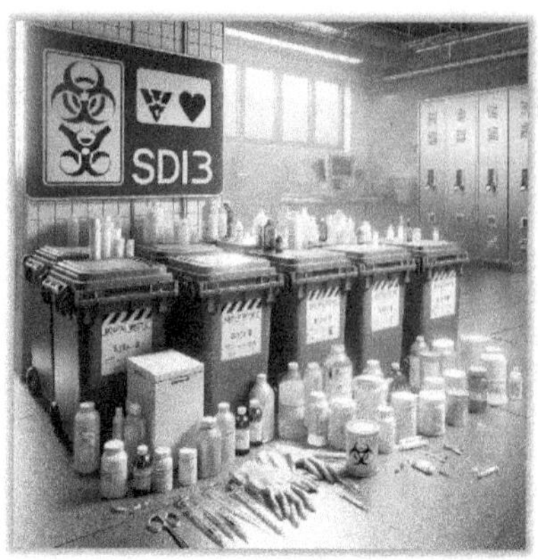


2. **Blood and Bodily Fluids:** Incidents such as accidents, violent crimes, and medical emergencies can expose individuals to bloodborne pathogens. Specialised cleaning and decontamination procedures are critical to ensure these sites are safe for public access.

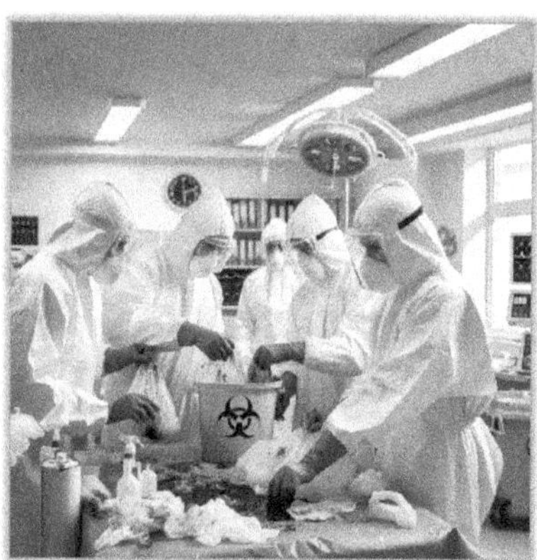

3. **Pathological Waste:** Tissues and fluids from medical procedures must be handled with the utmost care, requiring specific containment and disposal measures to prevent exposure to potentially infectious agents.

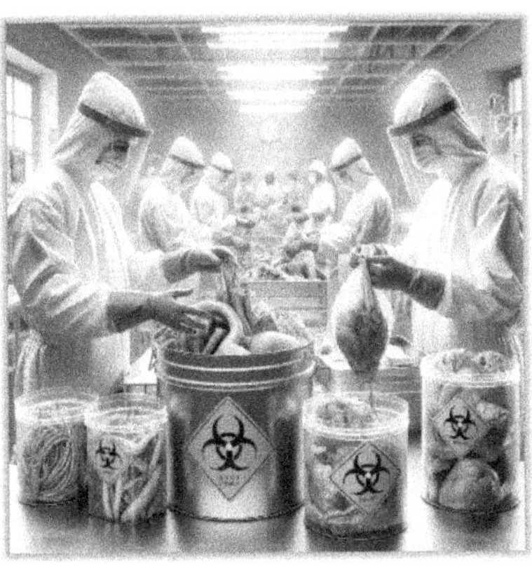

4. **Microbiological Wastes:** Research and diagnostic laboratories that work with infectious cultures, viral samples, and bacterial strains present unique challenges in preventing accidental releases or exposures.

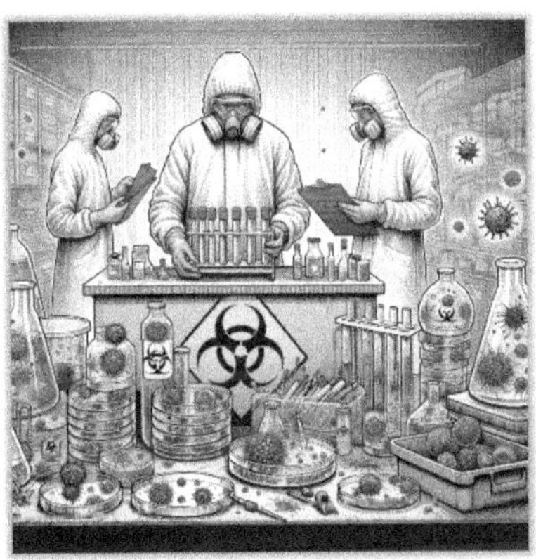

5. **Animal Waste:** Farms, veterinary clinics, and urban areas with significant wildlife populations can be sources of zoonotic diseases, necessitating proper waste management and sanitation practices.

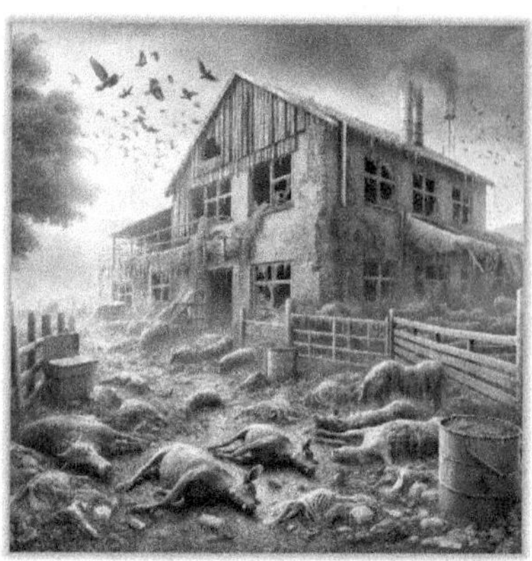

6. **Sewage and Faecal Matter:** The management of human and industrial waste is a public health priority, with the potential for widespread environmental contamination and disease transmission.

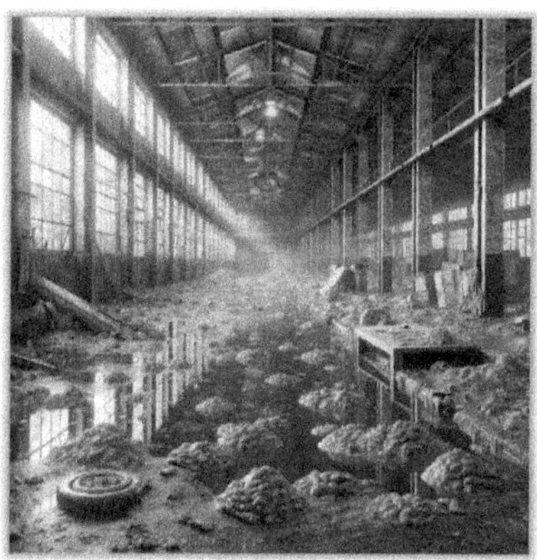

## Analysing Health and Environmental Impacts

The consequences of biohazard exposure extend beyond the immediate risk of infection or illness. Long-term health conditions, environmental degradation, and socio-economic impacts are critical considerations in the comprehensive management of biohazards.

- **Direct Health Impacts:** Exposure to biohazards can lead to acute and chronic illnesses, sometimes with long-lasting effects on the affected populations. The risk of outbreaks and the spread of infectious diseases necessitates robust public health responses.

- **Environmental Degradation:** Improper disposal or uncontrolled release of biohazards can lead to water, soil, and air pollution. This not only affects wildlife and ecosystems but also has a cascading effect on human health through the contamination of food and water supplies.

- **Socio-Economic Consequences:** The impact of biohazards on communities can be profound, affecting livelihoods, economic stability, and quality of life. The cost of remediation, healthcare, and lost productivity can place a significant burden on societies.

## The Imperative for Effective Biohazard Remediation

Addressing the challenges posed by biohazards requires a comprehensive strategy that encompasses identification, assessment, and the implementation of effective remediation techniques. This involves a multidisciplinary approach, engaging experts from the fields of microbiology, environmental science, public health, and emergency response.

**Strategic Approach to Biohazard Management**

- **Regulatory Compliance:** Adherence to legal and regulatory frameworks is foundational to effective biohazard management. This ensures that remediation efforts meet national standards and protect public health and the environment.

- **Technical Expertise:** The complexity of biohazard remediation demands specialised knowledge and skills. This includes understanding the nature of different biohazards, the appropriate use of disinfection and decontamination methods, and the implementation of safety protocols to protect remediation personnel and the public.

- **Innovation and Research:** Ongoing research and technological advancements are crucial for improving biohazard remediation techniques. Innovations in biohazard detection, containment, and neutralisation offer the potential for more effective and efficient responses to biohazard incidents.

- **Public Education and Awareness:** Informing the public about the risks associated with biohazards and the importance of prevention and proper disposal practices is essential for reducing the incidence and impact of biohazard exposures.

Understanding biohazards in the context of the UK involves grappling with a complex interplay of factors that influence human health and environmental safety. The diversity of biohazards, combined with the potential for widespread impacts, underscores the need for a comprehensive, informed, and proactive approach to their management and remediation.

# SECTION 2:
# LEGAL FRAMEWORK AND COMPLIANCE

The United Kingdom has established a comprehensive legal framework to govern the management and remediation of biohazards. This framework is designed to protect public health and the environment, ensuring that biohazardous materials are handled safely and effectively. Key regulations include:

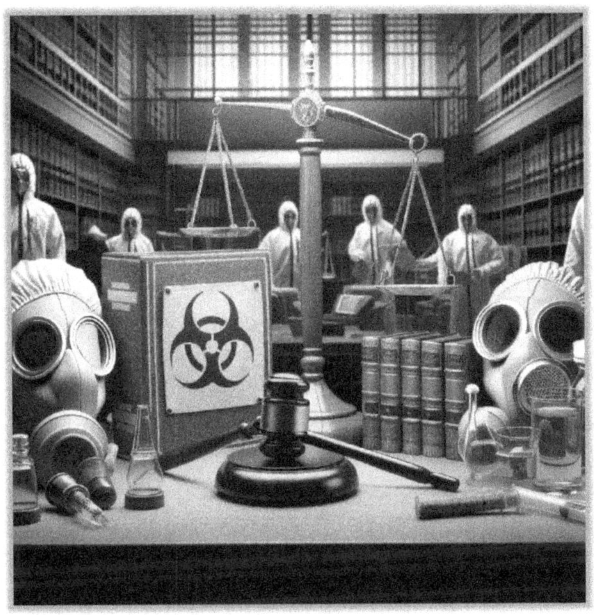

1. **Control of Substances Hazardous to Health Regulations (COSHH) 2002:** These regulations require employers to control substances that can be hazardous to health, including biohazards. Risk assessments, appropriate control measures, and training are mandated under COSHH.

2. **Health and Safety at Work etc. Act 1974:** This act places a duty on employers to ensure, as far as reasonably practicable, the health, safety, and welfare of their employees. This

includes providing a safe working environment during biohazard remediation.

3. **Environmental Protection Act 1990:** This act provides a framework for the proper management and disposal of waste, including hazardous waste, to protect the environment.

4. **Hazardous Waste (England and Wales) Regulations 2005:** These regulations specify how hazardous waste, including biohazardous waste, is to be managed, controlled, and disposed of.

5. **The Management of Health and Safety at Work Regulations 1999:** These regulations require employers to carry out risk assessments, make arrangements to implement necessary measures, appoint competent people, and arrange for appropriate information and training.

**Dutyholder Responsibilities and Compliance**

Dutyholder's, typically the employers or those in control of premises, have a legal obligation to comply with these regulations. Their responsibilities include:

1. **Conducting Risk Assessments:** Identifying potential biohazard risks and implementing measures to mitigate them.

2. **Implementing Control Measures:** Ensuring that appropriate safety measures, equipment, and procedures are in place.

3. **Providing Training and Information:** Educating employees about the risks associated with biohazards and the correct handling and remediation procedures.

4. **Safe Disposal of Biohazardous Waste:** Ensuring that biohazardous materials are disposed of in accordance with legal requirements.

5. **Record Keeping and Documentation:** Maintaining records of risk assessments, disposal certificates, and training sessions.

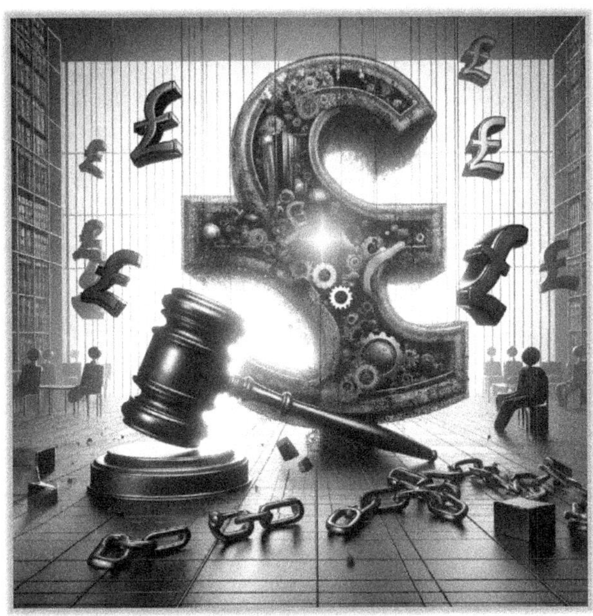

## Penalties for Non-Compliance

Failure to comply with these regulations can result in severe consequences, including:

1. **Fines:** Organisations can be fined for breaches of health and safety law. These fines can be substantial, reflecting the severity of the breach and the perceived risk to health.

2. **Prosecution:** In severe cases, dutyholder's can be prosecuted, which can lead to criminal convictions.

3. **Reputational Damage:** Non-compliance can lead to significant reputational harm, affecting business operations and relationships with clients and partners.

4. **Civil Claims:** Employers may face civil claims from employees or others affected by their failure to manage biohazards safely.

Compliance with these regulations is not just a legal requirement but also a moral and ethical obligation to protect the health and safety of employees, the public, and the environment. Understanding and adhering to these regulations is essential for all dutyholder's involved in biohazard remediation.

<h1 style="text-align:center">SECTION 3:<br>BIOHAZARD REMEDIATION PROCESS</h1>

The biohazard remediation process is a critical and multifaceted operation aimed at restoring safety and normalcy to environments contaminated with biological hazards. This process requires meticulous planning, rigorous safety measures, and stringent adherence to regulatory standards to effectively mitigate the risks posed by biohazards to health and the environment. Expanding upon the foundational steps outlined, we delve into a more comprehensive examination of each phase, underscoring the complexities and essential considerations that guide effective biohazard remediation.

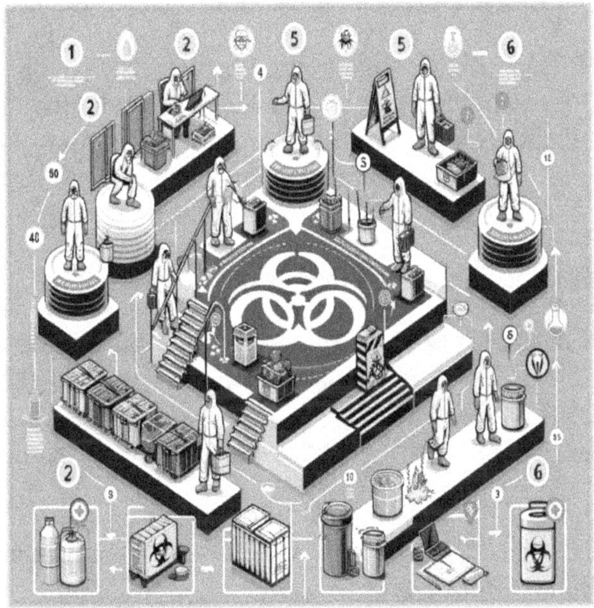

**Initial Assessment and Planning**

**1. Site Evaluation:** This initial step is crucial for understanding the scope of the biohazard situation. Specialists conduct a thorough inspection, using advanced tools and techniques to assess the extent of contamination. This may involve sampling and analysis to identify the types of biohazardous materials present and their concentrations, providing a basis for all subsequent remediation efforts.

**2. Risk Assessment:** A detailed risk assessment follows, identifying potential hazards to remediation workers, the public, and the environment. This assessment considers the nature of the biohazard, the likelihood of exposure, and the potential impact of exposure, facilitating the development of targeted safety measures.

**3. Remediation Plan:** Developing a comprehensive remediation plan is next, detailing the strategies, techniques, and resources required to safely and effectively address the biohazard. This plan includes specific procedures for decontamination, waste disposal, and site restoration, alongside timelines for execution and safety protocols to protect workers and the public.

**4. Communication:** Effective communication is established among all stakeholders, including remediation teams, clients, and relevant authorities. This ensures a coordinated approach, transparency, and compliance with regulatory requirements throughout the remediation process.

**Containment and Control Measures**

**1. Isolation of the Area:** Implementing physical barriers is essential to limit access to the contaminated area and contain the spread of biohazards. This may include fencing, signage, and the use of containment units or isolation chambers for highly infectious agents.

**2. Establishing Safety Zones:** Safety zones are created to delineate contaminated areas from those that are clean, ensuring a systematic and controlled approach to decontamination and minimising the risk of cross-contamination.

**3. Air Filtration and Ventilation Control:** Advanced air filtration systems and ventilation controls are employed to capture airborne contaminants and prevent their spread. This is particularly important in settings where biohazards can become aerosolised, posing an inhalation risk.

**4. Personal Protective Equipment (PPE):** The selection and use of appropriate PPE are critical to safeguard remediation workers. This includes respirators, gloves, protective suits, and eye protection, selected based on the specific biohazards and exposure risks involved.

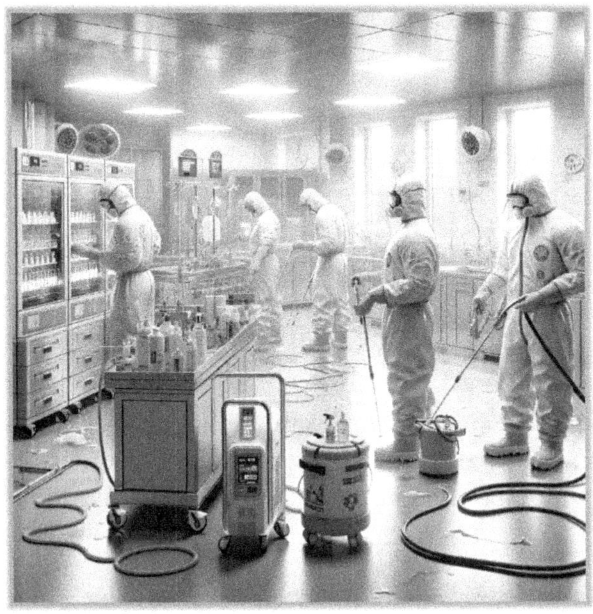

## Decontamination and Cleaning Procedures

**1. Removal of Contaminated Materials:** Contaminated materials are carefully removed and secured in biohazard bags for disposal. This step is performed with great caution to avoid disturbing the materials more than necessary, which could release pathogens into the environment.

**2. Cleaning and Sanitising:** All surfaces within the contaminated area are thoroughly cleaned using approved disinfectants, ensuring the elimination of biohazardous agents. This step may be repeated multiple times, depending on the level of contamination and the specific biohazards present.

**3. Verification of Decontamination:** Post-cleaning, rigorous testing is conducted to verify the absence of biohazards. This may include swab testing, air sampling, and other diagnostic assessments to ensure the area is safe for reoccupation.

**4. Restoration:** Finally, the area is restored to its original condition, which may involve structural repairs, repainting, and the replacement of fixtures and fittings. The goal is to return the space to a state that is safe, functional, and free from any reminder of the contamination.

**Waste Disposal and Management**

**1. Segregation and Labelling:** Biohazardous waste is segregated from other waste types and clearly labelled to ensure safe and compliant handling.

**2. Transportation:** Waste is transported in sealed, leak-proof containers to designated disposal facilities equipped to handle biohazardous materials safely.

**3. Compliant Disposal:** Disposal methods, such as autoclaving, incineration, or chemical disinfection, are carried out in accordance with legal and environmental regulations, ensuring the biohazard is neutralised.

**4. Documentation:** Detailed records of the disposal process are maintained, including the types of waste, quantities, disposal methods, and dates. This documentation is essential for regulatory compliance, tracking purposes, and providing assurance to clients and stakeholders that biohazards have been responsibly managed.

The biohazard remediation process is a comprehensive and highly specialised operation that demands expertise, precision, and a commitment to safety and environmental stewardship. Through these meticulously planned and executed steps, remediation professionals protect human health and the environment from the risks associated with biohazardous materials, restoring safety and peace of mind to affected communities.

# SPECIFIC TYPES OF BIOHAZARD CLEANING

Biohazard cleaning encompasses a wide array of specialised cleaning services designed to safely remove and dispose of biohazardous materials, ensuring environments are restored to safe, habitable conditions. The specifics of these services vary greatly depending on the nature of the biohazard, the environment affected, and the risks involved. Here, we expand on the various types of biohazard cleaning, offering deeper insights and additional examples to understand the complexity and necessity of each.

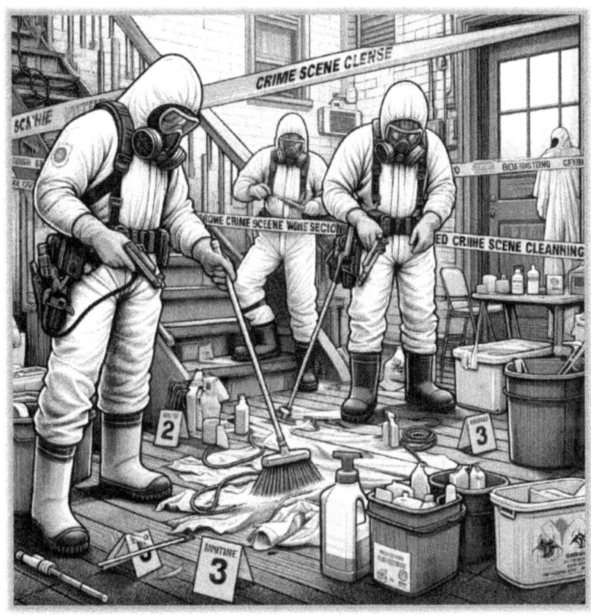


## Crime Scene Cleaning

Crime scene cleaning is one of the most recognised forms of biohazard remediation, often due to its portrayal in media. However, the reality is far more complex and sensitive. Professionals in this field are tasked with removing biological matter such as blood, tissue, and other bodily fluids that can carry pathogens like HIV, hepatitis B, and hepatitis C.

- **Suicide and Homicide Cleanup:** Beyond the removal of biological matter, these situations often require dealing with the emotional distress of the affected families, requiring cleaners to work with compassion and sensitivity.

- **Chemical Treatment:** Specialised chemicals, often hospital-grade disinfectants, are used to ensure complete neutralisation of pathogens. These may include products capable of breaking down bloodborne pathogens on a molecular level.

- **Restoration:** Often involves repairing or replacing flooring, drywall, and furnishings, sometimes extending to structural elements damaged during the incident or the investigation.

## Trauma and Blood/Bodily Fluid Cleaning

Trauma scenes extend beyond crime scenes to include accidents, industrial injuries, and natural deaths, where significant biohazard contamination can occur.

- **Accident Scenes:** Industrial or vehicular accidents can spread biohazardous materials over large areas and diverse surfaces, requiring extensive containment measures.

- **Sanitisation Techniques:** Use of ultraviolet light for sanitising areas that are hard to reach with traditional cleaning methods.

- **Deodorisation:** Often requires multiple treatments, including ozone generators to neutralise odours that cleaning alone cannot remove.

## Animal Waste and Hoarding Cleaning

These scenarios can pose unique challenges, combining biohazard removal with the need to address severe clutter and damage to properties.

- **Severe Hoarding Situations:** Can involve not just animal waste but also decaying food, pests, and mould, requiring a multi-faceted cleaning and sanitisation approach.

- **Sanitisation:** Involves deep cleaning techniques and the use of enzyme treatments to break down waste materials and eliminate odours at the source.

- **Odor Control:** May require the sealing of surfaces or the use of advanced air scrubbing technology to fully remove odours.

## Unattended Death and Drug Paraphernalia Cleaning

Unattended deaths can lead to significant biological hazard scenarios, particularly if the body has been decomposing for an extended period. Drug paraphernalia adds an additional layer of risk due to the potential for sharp objects and exposure to harmful substances.

- **Decomposition Cleanup:** Requires special attention to fluids that have penetrated flooring or walls, often necessitating structural removal and replacement.

- **Disinfection:** Utilisation of broad-spectrum disinfectants and, in some cases, fogging techniques to ensure comprehensive treatment of the area.

- **Safe Handling:** Implementing procedures for the safe collection and disposal of sharps and ensuring that drug residues are fully eradicated.

**Sewage/Faeces Cleaning**

Sewage backups and faecal contaminations are biohazard scenarios fraught with bacteria, viruses, and parasites that can cause serious health issues.

- **Flood Restoration:** Following natural disasters, cleaning efforts may involve addressing contamination from sewage that has infiltrated homes.

- **Disinfection and Cleaning:** High-pressure washing combined with antimicrobial treatments to sanitise affected areas thoroughly.

- **Mould Prevention:** Strategic drying and humidity control measures to prevent mould growth, often using industrial dehumidifiers and air movers.

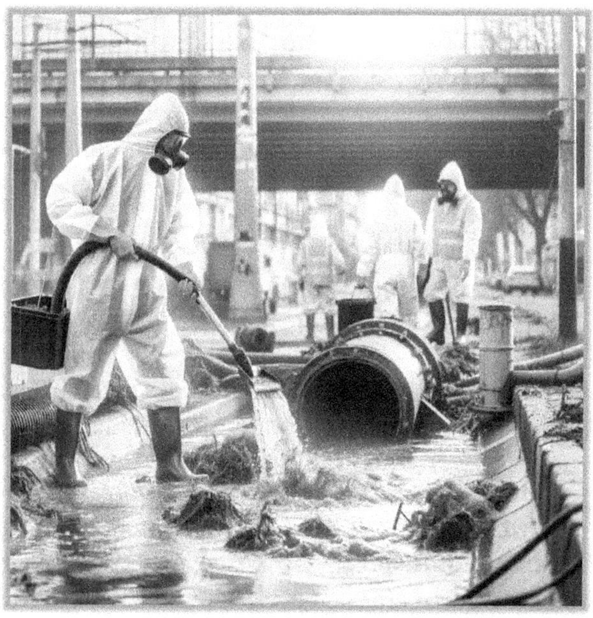

## Infectious Disease Cleanup

The outbreak of infectious diseases, whether in a residential, commercial, or healthcare setting, requires rigorous cleaning protocols to prevent the spread of illness.

- **Pandemic Response:** COVID-19 highlighted the need for rapid response teams capable of disinfecting facilities exposed to the virus, using electrostatic sprayers to apply disinfectants.

- **High-Level Disinfection:** Techniques may include the use of autoclaves for sterilising equipment or heat treatments for spaces where chemical sensitivities are a concern.

- **PPE Usage:** Ensuring the latest in protective gear is used, adapting to the nature of the infectious agent, to protect cleaning crews while minimising the risk of cross-contamination.

Each type of biohazard cleaning demands a high level of expertise, specialised equipment, and a deep understanding of the risks involved. Professionals in this field not only restore environments to their original state but also ensure the safety and well-being of individuals affected by these traumatic events, highlighting the critical role biohazard cleaning plays in public health and safety.

# SECTION 5:
# CHOOSING THE RIGHT REMEDIATION COMPANY

Choosing the right biohazard remediation company is a crucial decision that impacts the safety, efficacy, and compliance of the cleanup process. The selection process involves a comprehensive evaluation of the company's qualifications, the technologies they employ, their commitment to industry standards, and their proven experience in the field. Here's a deeper dive into the essential criteria for selecting a biohazard remediation company, without specific examples but with a clear explanation of each factor's importance.

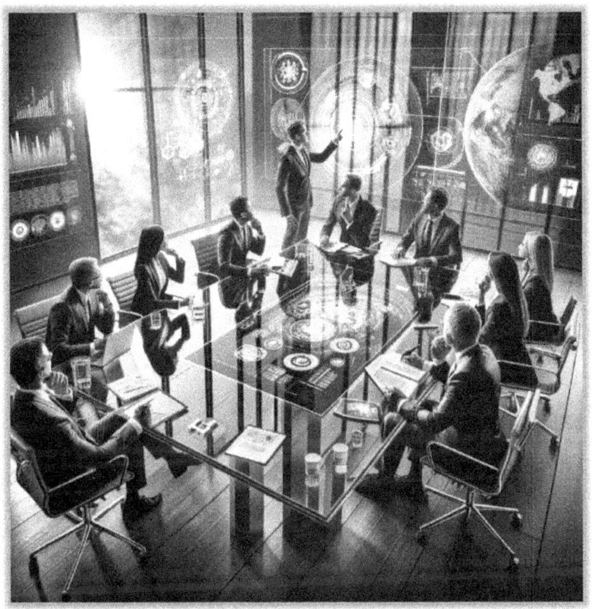

## Professional Training

The foundation of a capable remediation team lies in its comprehensive training regimen. This training should cover the full spectrum of biohazard remediation, including the safe handling of hazardous materials, the correct use of decontamination chemicals, and adherence to safety protocols. Accreditation by reputable organisations ensures that staff are well-equipped to manage biohazard scenarios effectively.

## Certification

Certifications from recognised industry bodies serve as proof of an individual's expertise and the company's dedication to excellence. These credentials indicate a professional's ability to meet rigorous standards in biohazard cleanup and remediation, ensuring quality and safety in their work.

## Continuous Education

The field of biohazard remediation is continuously evolving. Companies that prioritise ongoing education for their staff ensure that their teams are updated with the latest practices, technological advancements, and regulatory changes, maintaining their effectiveness and compliance.

## Advanced Equipment

The complexity of biohazard remediation necessitates the use of advanced equipment for cleaning, sanitising, and air filtration. High-quality tools not only enhance the effectiveness of the cleanup process but also ensure it is completed safely and efficiently.

## Safety Gear

The personal safety of remediation workers is paramount. Companies must provide their staff with high-quality personal protective equipment (PPE), including respirators, gloves, and protective suits, to safeguard them against exposure to hazardous materials.

## Technological Sophistication

Employing the latest technological solutions for risk assessment, monitoring, and reporting can significantly improve the remediation process's efficiency and transparency. These technologies enable precise hazard identification, continuous monitoring, and comprehensive documentation for regulatory compliance.

## Industry Certifications

Affiliation with and certifications from recognised bodies underscore a company's commitment to quality, safety, and adherence to best practices. This is crucial for maintaining high standards in biohazard remediation work.

## Compliance with Standards

Adhering to national and international standards ensures that remediation work meets the highest safety and quality levels. This commitment is essential for upholding safe environments for workers and the public alike.

## Regulatory Adherence

Staying compliant with local, regional, and national regulations is critical to ensure that biohazardous materials are handled, treated, and disposed of properly. This minimises environmental impact and public health risks, ensuring responsible remediation practices.

## Years in Business

The length of time a company has been operational can provide insight into its experience and reliability. Longer-standing companies are likely to have managed a diverse array of biohazard situations, reflecting a depth of knowledge and expertise.

## Past Projects

Reviewing a company's history of projects offers a glimpse into its capacity to handle specific biohazard scenarios. This includes its adaptability to different challenges and its effectiveness in various situations.

## Client Testimonials and Reviews

Feedback from previous clients can shed light on a company's professionalism, efficiency, and customer service quality. Positive reviews are strong indicators of a company's reputation for satisfactory and reliable service.

## Case Studies

Case studies of past remediation projects can offer detailed insights into a company's approach to problem-solving and its success in managing complex remediation tasks. This demonstrates the company's strategic planning, execution, and ability to restore safety effectively.

In choosing a biohazard remediation company, stakeholders must carefully assess these factors to ensure the selected provider is capable of delivering safe, effective, and compliant biohazard remediation services. This careful consideration ensures that the remediation process is conducted with the highest standards of safety and professionalism, safeguarding public health and the environment.

# SECTION 6:
# BEST PRACTICES IN BIOHAZARD REMEDIATION

Best practices in biohazard remediation are critical to ensuring the safety and health of both the remediation team and the public, while also preserving the integrity and confidentiality of the affected areas. These practices are foundational to the professional and ethical execution of biohazard cleanup tasks, which can range from dealing with infectious disease outbreaks to cleaning up after a crime scene. The complexity and potential danger of these tasks necessitate a comprehensive approach that encompasses risk assessment, the use of personal protective equipment (PPE), adherence to safety protocols, and a commitment to ethical and discreet cleaning practices.

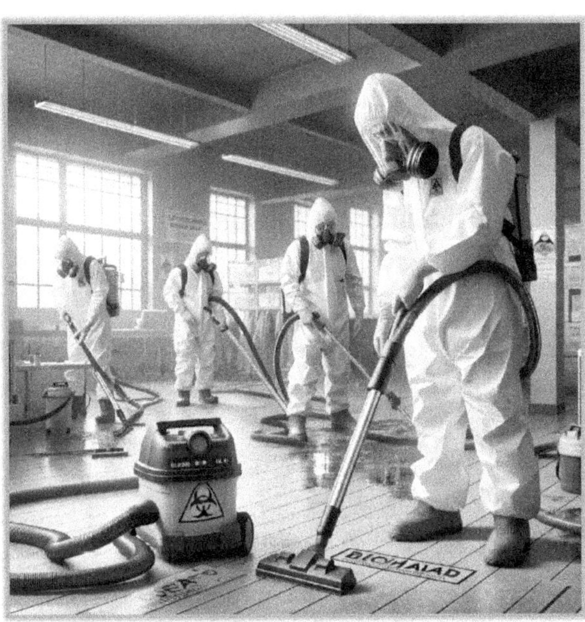

**Risk Assessment**

The first step in any biohazard remediation project is a thorough risk assessment. This process involves identifying the types of biohazards present, understanding the potential routes of exposure, and assessing the risk to all individuals involved, including remediation workers, clients, and the general public. A detailed risk assessment informs the development of a tailored remediation plan that addresses the specific hazards of the situation.

- **Dynamic Risk Assessment:** This ongoing process allows for the continuous evaluation of risks as the remediation progresses, adapting strategies in response to new information or changes in the environment.

**Use of Personal Protective Equipment (PPE)**

The use of appropriate PPE is non-negotiable in biohazard remediation. Equipment such as gloves, masks, respirators, and protective suits create barriers against infectious agents, chemicals, and other hazardous materials encountered during cleanup.

- **PPE Training:** Workers must not only have access to high-quality PPE but also be trained in its proper use, including how to correctly put on, take off, dispose of, and maintain this equipment to prevent contamination.

**Safety Protocols**

Implementing and enforcing strict safety protocols ensures the effective management of biohazards, protecting both workers and the public. These protocols cover a range of practices, from the secure containment and removal of biohazardous materials to the decontamination of affected areas.

- **Emergency Response Plans:** Detailed plans for handling unexpected incidents or exposures during remediation activities are essential for maintaining safety and minimising risks.

## Client Protection

Protecting clients and the public involves not only physical safety measures but also clear communication about the risks and the steps being taken to mitigate those risks. Securing the remediation area to prevent unauthorised access and providing regular updates to clients are key components of this practice.

- **Community Engagement:** In cases where broader communities may be affected, engaging with community leaders and the public to address concerns and provide reassurance is crucial.

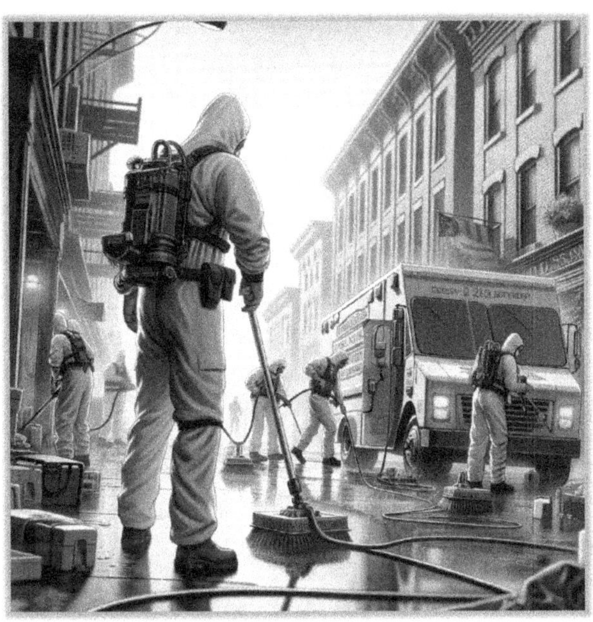

## Ethical and Discreet Cleaning Practices

Given the often sensitive nature of biohazard remediation, ethical and discreet practices are paramount. Maintaining the confidentiality of the clients and the situation, treating all involved with empathy and respect, and conducting cleanup operations discreetly to avoid unnecessary attention are fundamental.

- **Cultural Sensitivity:** Understanding and respecting cultural and personal values related to death, trauma, and property is essential for conducting biohazard remediation with compassion and respect.

## Quality Control and Assurance

High standards of quality in biohazard remediation not only ensure the safety and efficacy of the cleanup but also build trust with clients. Adhering to standard operating procedures, conducting regular quality checks, and maintaining detailed documentation are all critical for achieving these standards.

- **Third-Party Certifications:** Obtaining certifications from industry-recognised bodies can provide an objective measure of a company's commitment to quality and safety standards.

## Continuous Improvement and Training

The field of biohazard remediation is constantly evolving, driven by advances in science, technology, and industry best practices. Committing to continuous improvement and training ensures that remediation teams are always equipped with the latest knowledge and tools to effectively handle biohazard situations.

- **Innovation:** Actively seeking out and incorporating new cleaning agents, equipment, and methodologies can enhance the efficiency and effectiveness of biohazard remediation, reducing risks and improving outcomes.

## Feedback and Evaluation

Utilising feedback from clients and conducting post-job evaluations are invaluable for identifying areas of improvement and celebrating successes. This feedback loop supports ongoing learning and development within the remediation team.

- **Case Studies:** Analysing completed projects to extract lessons learned and best practices not only improves future remediation efforts but also contributes to the broader body of knowledge in the field.

**Research and Development**

Staying at the forefront of the biohazard remediation field requires active engagement in research and development. This can involve collaborating with academic institutions, industry groups, and regulatory agencies to develop safer, more effective cleanup methods and technologies.

- **Partnerships:** Building partnerships with research organisations and other stakeholders can facilitate the exchange of knowledge and resources, driving innovation in biohazard remediation techniques and equipment.

Best practices in biohazard remediation encompass a broad spectrum of activities and principles, from initial risk assessment and the use of PPE to ethical cleaning practices, quality assurance, and a commitment to continuous improvement. By adhering to these practices, biohazard remediation professionals not only ensure the safety and well-being of themselves and those they serve but also uphold the highest standards of professionalism and care in their work.

# SECTION 7:
# AFTERMATH AND RESTORATION

The aftermath of a biohazard incident and the subsequent restoration process are critical phases that extend well beyond the initial cleanup and decontamination efforts. These steps are essential not only for restoring the physical environment but also for addressing the psychological impacts on those affected. The comprehensive approach to aftermath and restoration involves meticulous testing for safety, property repair, and providing psychological support, each of which plays a vital role in the holistic recovery process.

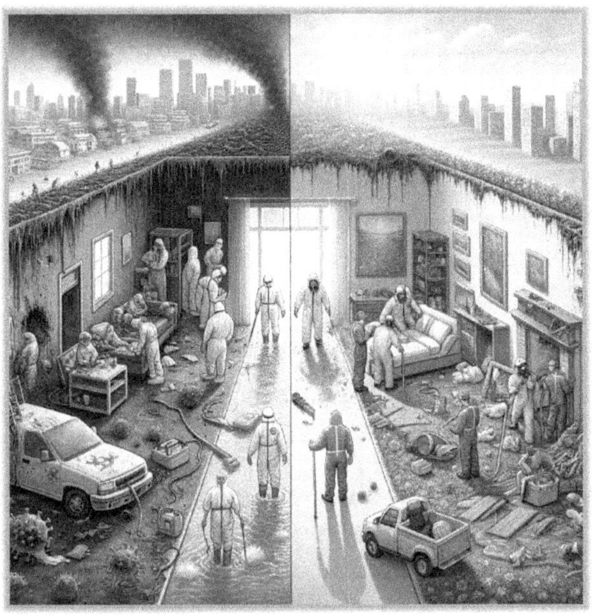

## Testing for Residual Contaminants

After decontamination, rigorous testing for residual contaminants is imperative to ensure the environment is safe for reoccupation. This phase involves:

- **Swab Testing and Air Quality Assessments:** These tests are designed to detect the presence of biohazards at a microbial level, ensuring no pathogens remain that could pose health risks. Air quality assessments are particularly important in cases where airborne pathogens or toxic chemicals were involved.

- **Laboratory Analyses:** Samples collected during testing are analysed in specialised laboratories equipped to detect a wide range of biological and chemical contaminants. This scientific analysis provides a quantitative measure of the cleanup's effectiveness.

- **Continuous Monitoring:** In some situations, ongoing monitoring of the environment may be necessary to ensure that the area remains safe over time, especially in cases where there is a risk of recontamination.

## Validation of Cleaning Procedures

Validating the cleaning procedures involves a thorough review of the methods and protocols used during remediation to ensure they align with industry standards and best practices. This step is crucial for:

- **Ensuring Compliance:** Validation confirms that all cleaning and decontamination efforts have adhered to regulatory requirements and guidelines specific to biohazard remediation.

- **Benchmarking Against Protocols:** It involves comparing the cleaning processes used against established protocols to identify any deviations or areas for improvement.

## Certification of Safety

Issuing a certification of safety is the final step in affirming that the area is free from biohazards and safe for occupants. This certification:

- **Provides Peace of Mind:** For property owners, occupants, and the surrounding community, knowing the area has been certified safe is crucial for peace of mind and confidence in returning to normal activities.

- **Ensures Legal Compliance:** The certification serves as documentation of compliance with health and safety regulations, which can be important for insurance purposes and potential legal considerations.

## Property Restoration and Repair

The physical restoration of the property addresses the structural and aesthetic damage caused by the biohazard and the remediation process. This phase includes:

- **Damage Assessment:** A comprehensive evaluation of the property to identify all areas impacted by the biohazard, assessing both visible damage and potential structural issues that may not be immediately apparent.

- **Restoration Work:** Depending on the extent of the damage, restoration can range from simple cleaning and painting to complete reconstruction of affected areas. This work aims to return the property to its pre-incident condition or better.

- **Coordination with Specialists:** The restoration process often requires the expertise of various professionals, including contractors, electricians, plumbers, and interior designers, to ensure all aspects of the property are appropriately addressed.

## Psychological Support and Counselling Resources

The emotional and psychological impact of biohazard incidents on individuals can be profound and long-lasting. Addressing these impacts is an essential part of the restoration process:

- **Recognising Emotional Impact:** Acknowledging the psychological trauma associated with biohazard incidents, especially those involving violence, death, or significant disruption to daily life, is the first step in providing support.

- **Referral to Support Services:** Offering referrals to counselling and mental health services provides those affected with access to professional support and coping strategies. This may include individual therapy, group counselling, or specialised services for trauma.

- **Community Resources:** Connecting individuals with community support groups and resources can offer additional layers of support, fostering a sense of solidarity and shared recovery among those affected.

The aftermath and restoration phase following a biohazard incident are multifaceted, encompassing not only the physical cleaning and repair of the property but also the safety verification and emotional support for those impacted. This holistic approach ensures that all aspects of recovery are addressed, facilitating a return to normalcy while safeguarding the health and well-being of individuals and the community at large.

# SECTION 8:
# CASE STUDIES AND REAL-WORLD EXAMPLES

The realm of biohazard remediation encompasses a wide array of scenarios, each presenting unique challenges and requiring specialised solutions. Through an examination of case studies and real-world examples, we can gain a deeper understanding of the intricacies involved in effectively managing and mitigating biohazard incidents. Additionally, insights from industry experts further enrich our understanding, shedding light on the evolving landscape of biohazard remediation. This comprehensive analysis aims to underscore the critical importance of preparedness, adaptability, and continuous learning in the field.

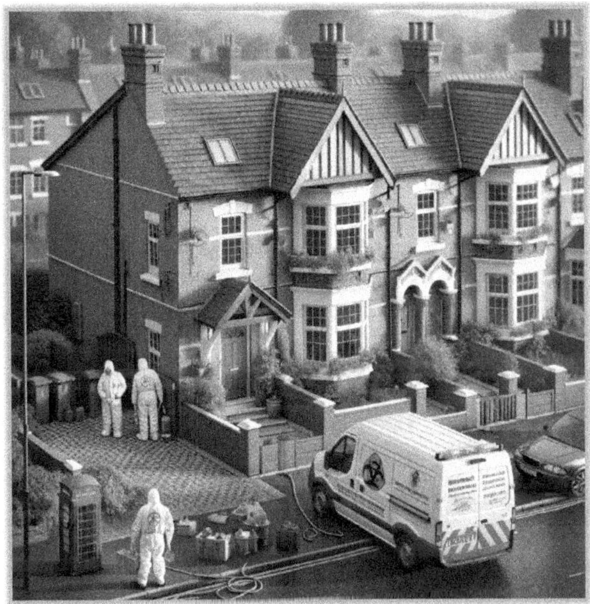

## Case Study 1: Crime Scene Cleanup

A residential neighbourhood was rocked by a tragic incident that resulted in a homicide within a family home. The remediation team faced the challenge of not only cleaning the physical remnants of the crime but also doing so with sensitivity to the emotional trauma experienced by the family and community.

**Challenges Faced:**

- Removal of biological contaminants, including blood and tissue, while preserving the integrity of the crime scene for investigative purposes.

- Providing emotional support to the grieving family and ensuring the cleanup process was handled discreetly and respectfully.

**Solutions Implemented:**

- Collaboration with the police to ensure that cleaning efforts did not compromise evidence.

- Use of advanced biohazard cleaning technologies to thoroughly decontaminate the scene.

- Implementation of discreet cleanup practices to maintain the family's privacy.

**Outcomes Achieved:**

- The property was restored to a safe and habitable condition, allowing the family to begin the healing process.

- The cleanup team was commended for their professionalism and empathy, highlighting the importance of sensitivity in crime scene cleanup operations.

**Case Study 2: Infectious Disease Decontamination**

An outbreak of a highly contagious virus in a large office building prompted an urgent response from biohazard remediation specialists SRS. The team was tasked with decontaminating the building to prevent further spread of the disease.

**Challenges Faced:**

- Implementing a decontamination plan that was thorough yet efficient to minimise downtime for the business.

- Ensuring the safety of the remediation team while working in an environment with a high risk of exposure.

**Solutions Implemented:**

- Use of electrostatic sprayers to apply disinfectants evenly across surfaces, ensuring comprehensive coverage.

- Adoption of stringent PPE protocols to protect remediation workers from exposure.

**Outcomes Achieved:**

- The building was successfully decontaminated, with no subsequent cases of the virus reported among the building's occupants.

- The business was able to resume operations with minimal disruption, underscoring the efficacy of rapid response and advanced decontamination techniques.

### Case Study 3: Large-Scale Industrial Accident

A chemical spill at an industrial facility resulted in widespread contamination, posing serious health risks to workers and the surrounding environment.

**Challenges Faced:**

- Containing the spill to prevent further environmental damage.

- Safely cleaning and neutralising a wide range of hazardous chemicals.

**Solutions Implemented:**

- Deployment of environmental containment measures, including barriers and absorbent materials, to limit the spread of contaminants.

- Utilisation of chemical neutralisation techniques tailored to the specific substances involved in the spill.

**Outcomes Achieved:**

- The spill was successfully contained and neutralised, preventing long-term environmental impact.

- The incident prompted a review and enhancement of safety protocols at the facility, reducing the risk of future accidents.

**Interviews with Industry Experts**

Insights from seasoned industry experts provide additional depth to our understanding of biohazard remediation. One SRS expert highlighted the critical role of technology in enhancing the speed and efficacy of cleanup operations, pointing to the growing use of robotics and automation to safely handle hazardous materials. Another emphasised the importance of mental health support for remediation workers, who often face traumatic scenes in the line of duty. Providing access to counselling and support services was identified as a key factor in maintaining a resilient workforce.

Future trends in the industry are pointing towards increased regulation and standardisation of biohazard remediation practices. Experts anticipate a greater emphasis on sustainability and environmental responsibility in cleanup operations, driven by public awareness and regulatory pressures.

<h1 style="text-align:center">SECTION 9:<br>FUTURE TRENDS AND INNOVATIONS</h1>

The future of biohazard remediation is poised at the brink of revolutionary change, driven by technological innovation, legislative evolution, and a dynamic shift in best practices. This evolution promises not only to transform the methods and tools available for biohazard cleanup but also to redefine the standards of safety, efficiency, and environmental stewardship within the industry. As we look ahead, it's clear that the field will increasingly rely on advanced technologies, stringent regulatory frameworks, and an integrated approach to remediation that prioritises both environmental and human health.

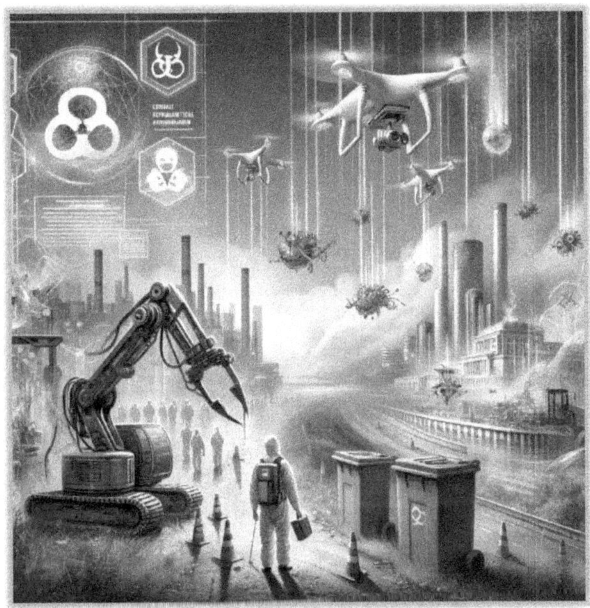

## Technological Advancements in Biohazard Remediation

The advent of robotic cleaning devices marks a significant leap forward in biohazard remediation. These robots, equipped with sensors and cleaning tools, can enter areas that are too dangerous for human teams, such as zones with high levels of toxic chemicals or radiation. Their precision and ability to operate in hazardous conditions minimise human exposure to biohazards and enhance the safety of the remediation process.

Drones, too, are set to play a pivotal role in the industry. Capable of flying over and mapping contaminated areas, drones can quickly assess the extent of a biohazard spill, identify hotspots of contamination, and even deliver remediation agents to specific areas. This aerial perspective not only speeds up the assessment process but also improves the accuracy of contamination mapping, allowing for targeted and efficient cleanup efforts.

The field is also witnessing the emergence of advanced bioremediation techniques that harness the power of microorganisms to break down and neutralise biohazards naturally. These techniques offer an eco-friendly alternative to chemical decontaminants, reducing the environmental footprint of remediation projects. Moreover, the development of nanotechnology-based solutions, including nanoparticles that can bind to and neutralise pathogens, is set to enhance the effectiveness of decontamination efforts while minimising harm to the environment.

**Legislative and Regulatory Updates**

As our understanding of biohazards and their impacts deepens, legislative and regulatory frameworks are evolving to ensure that remediation practices keep pace with scientific and technological advancements. Future legislative updates are expected to focus on tightening safety standards, mandating more rigorous training and certification for remediation personnel, and enhancing transparency and accountability throughout the remediation process.

Professionals in the field must stay informed about these changes to ensure compliance and safeguard public health. Anticipated regulatory shifts may include stricter guidelines for handling specific types of biohazards, such as emerging infectious diseases or chemical spills, and increased requirements for documenting and reporting remediation efforts. These changes aim to standardise remediation practices, ensuring a high level of protection for workers, the public, and the environment.

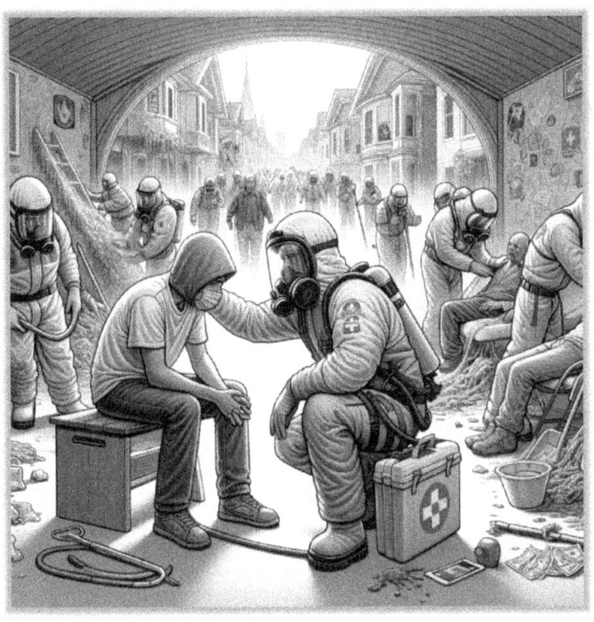

## Evolving Best Practices

The best practices in biohazard remediation are evolving to reflect a more holistic approach to cleanup efforts. This includes recognising the psychological and social impacts of biohazard incidents, in addition to addressing the physical aspects of cleanup. Future trends in best practices are likely to emphasise the need for remediation teams to be trained in psychological first aid, enabling them to support affected individuals and communities more effectively.

The development of international standards for biohazard remediation is another key trend. These standards will facilitate global collaboration and knowledge sharing, ensuring that remediation efforts worldwide adhere to the highest levels of safety and effectiveness. Additionally, the integration of continuous improvement frameworks into remediation practices will encourage ongoing learning and adaptation, driving the industry towards more effective, efficient, and compassionate outcomes.

Increased collaboration across industries, including healthcare, emergency services, and environmental protection, will also shape the future of biohazard remediation. By working together, these sectors can develop comprehensive strategies for managing biohazard incidents, from initial response to long-term recovery, ensuring that all aspects of public health and safety are addressed.

The future of biohazard remediation is marked by exciting technological innovations, evolving legislative and regulatory landscapes, and a shift towards more integrated and holistic best practices. These developments promise to enhance the safety, efficiency, and environmental sustainability of remediation efforts, ultimately leading to more effective responses to biohazard incidents and better protection for public health and the environment. As the field continues to evolve, professionals must remain agile, informed, and committed to adopting these advancements to meet the challenges of biohazard remediation in the 21st century and beyond.

# SECTION 10:
# RESOURCES AND SUPPORT

Navigating the complexities of biohazard remediation requires more than just technical skills and equipment; it demands a deep understanding of the regulatory environment, safety standards, and the latest advancements in the field. Access to a comprehensive suite of resources and support mechanisms is indispensable for professionals committed to excellence in biohazard remediation. This detailed exploration delves into the various resources available to those in the industry, highlighting the importance of regulatory bodies, professional associations, and educational materials in enhancing professional practice.

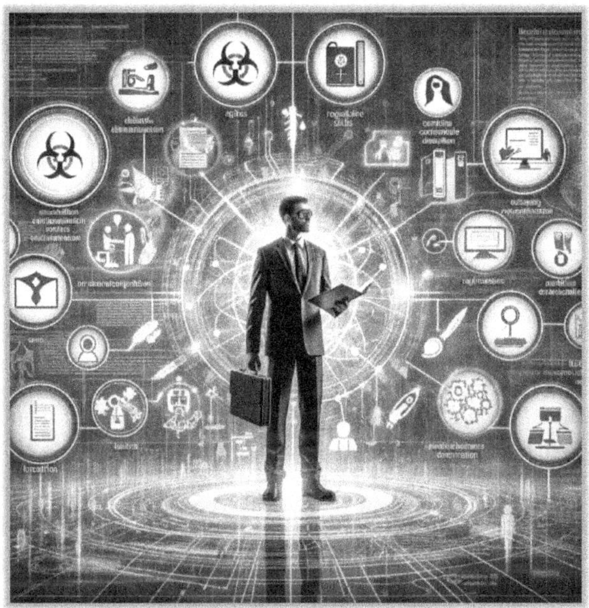

## Government and Industry Resources

The backbone of effective biohazard remediation lies in adherence to guidelines and regulations set forth by authoritative entities. Regulatory bodies such as the Environmental Protection Agency (EPA) in the United States, the Health and Safety Executive (HSE) in the United Kingdom, and similar organisations worldwide, play a pivotal role in establishing the standards for safe and effective biohazard management. These agencies offer a wealth of resources, including:

- **Regulatory Guidelines:** Comprehensive documents outlining the legal requirements for handling various biohazards, from chemical spills to infectious disease outbreaks. These guidelines serve as a roadmap for ensuring compliance during remediation projects.

- **Safety Protocols:** Detailed protocols for the safe handling, transportation, and disposal of biohazardous materials, aimed at protecting both remediation professionals and the public.

- **Advisory Documents:** Best practice advisories that offer insights into the most effective approaches for biohazard cleanup, based on the latest scientific research and industry standards.

Access to these resources ensures that professionals are equipped with the knowledge to navigate the legal and practical challenges of biohazard remediation, ensuring safety and compliance across all operations.

**Professional Associations and Networks**

Professional associations are instrumental in fostering a culture of continuous improvement and excellence within the biohazard remediation industry. By joining organisations such as the American Bio-Recovery Association (ABRA), the Institute of Inspection, Cleaning and Restoration Certification (IICRC), or the British Institute of Cleaning Science (BICSc), professionals gain access to:

- **Certification Programs:** Rigorous training and certification programs that validate a professional's expertise in biohazard remediation, enhancing their credibility and marketability.

- **Continuing Education:** Opportunities for ongoing learning through workshops, seminars, and conferences that cover the latest developments and challenges in the field.

- **Networking Opportunities:** Platforms for connecting with peers, sharing experiences, and collaborating on best practices, fostering a community of shared knowledge and support.

Membership in these associations not only signals a commitment to the highest standards of professional practice but also provides invaluable resources for personal and organisational development.

**Further Reading and Educational Materials**

For those keen on deepening their expertise in biohazard remediation, a wealth of educational materials is available. Books such as "Biohazard Cleanup: Procedures and Practices" offer comprehensive insights into the technical aspects of remediation, while peer-reviewed articles in journals like the "Journal of Environmental Health" and "Infection Control and Hospital Epidemiology" provide the latest research findings and innovative approaches to biohazard management. Additionally, case studies of real-world remediation projects can offer practical insights into the challenges and solutions encountered by professionals in the field.

Online courses and webinars, offered by educational institutions and industry associations, cover a broad spectrum of topics, including:

- **Technical Cleaning Protocols:** Detailed instruction on the methods and materials used in biohazard remediation, tailored to specific types of biohazards.

- **Health and Safety Management:** Guidance on creating and implementing effective safety management systems for biohazard remediation operations.

- **Psychological Aspects of Trauma Cleaning:** Training on the emotional and psychological considerations of working in environments affected by trauma, providing strategies for supporting affected individuals and communities.

These resources not only enhance the technical skills of biohazard remediation professionals but also broaden their understanding of the wider implications of their work, including the environmental, psychological, and community impacts.

In conclusion, the field of biohazard remediation is supported by a rich array of resources and support mechanisms designed to promote safety, compliance, and professional excellence. By leveraging these resources, professionals can stay informed about the latest developments in the field, enhance their operational capabilities, and ultimately contribute to safer and more effective biohazard remediation practices. This commitment to continuous learning and adherence to industry standards is essential for addressing the complex challenges posed by biohazard incidents and ensuring the health and safety of both workers and the broader community.

# GLOBAL PERSPECTIVES AND INTERNATIONAL COOPERATION

The management of biohazard incidents transcends national boundaries, necessitating a coordinated global response to effectively mitigate risks and protect public health and the environment. The complexity and unpredictability of biohazards, ranging from pandemics to chemical spills, underscore the importance of international cooperation and the development of unified standards and protocols for biohazard remediation.

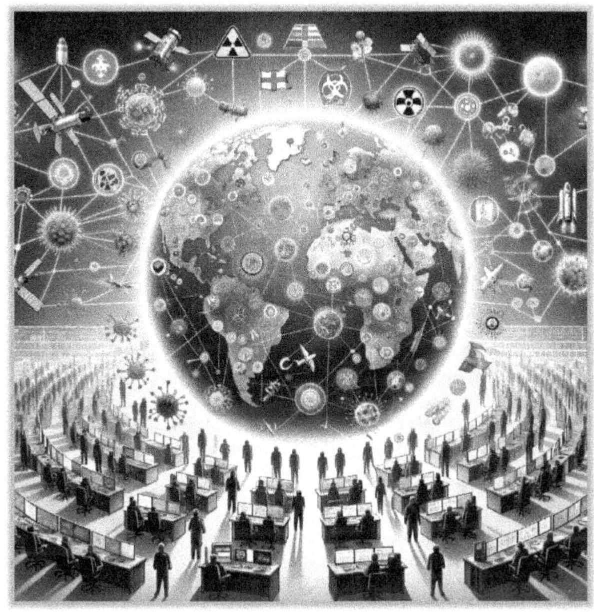

## International Biohazard Management

The global nature of biohazard risks is evident in the rapid spread of infectious diseases, the international trade of potentially hazardous materials, and the environmental impacts of industrial accidents that can affect multiple countries. Global health organisations, such as the World Health Organisation (WHO) and the Centres for Disease Control and Prevention (CDC), play pivotal roles in coordinating responses to biohazard incidents. These organisations facilitate the sharing of information, resources, and best practices among countries, helping to build a comprehensive and effective global biohazard management strategy.

**International cooperation in biohazard management involves:**

- **Surveillance and Early Warning Systems:** Implementing global networks for disease surveillance and early warning systems that can detect and report outbreaks promptly.

- **Resource Sharing:** Mobilising and sharing resources, including vaccines, medical supplies, and remediation equipment, to areas impacted by biohazard incidents.

- **Joint Research Initiatives:** Collaborating on research initiatives to better understand biohazards and develop innovative remediation technologies and methodologies.

**Case Studies of International Biohazard Response**

Several case studies highlight the effectiveness of international cooperation in responding to biohazard incidents:

- **The Ebola Outbreak in West Africa (2014-2016):** An international response, coordinated by the WHO and supported by multiple countries and NGOs, was crucial in containing the outbreak. The deployment of international medical teams, the provision of emergency supplies, and the implementation of public health measures helped to control the spread of the disease.

- **The Chernobyl Nuclear Disaster (1986):** The Chernobyl disaster prompted a global response to address the nuclear fallout that affected several countries in Europe. International teams of experts were involved in the containment and cleanup efforts, and the incident led to the establishment of international safety standards for nuclear power plants.

- **The COVID-19 Pandemic:** The ongoing global effort to manage the COVID-19 pandemic exemplifies international cooperation, with countries sharing information on the virus, collaborating on the development and distribution of vaccines, and implementing coordinated public health measures to mitigate the spread of the disease.

These case studies underscore the value of collaborative efforts in addressing complex biohazard incidents, demonstrating that international cooperation is essential for effective biohazard management.

**Global Standards and Protocols**

The development and implementation of international standards and protocols for biohazard remediation are critical for ensuring a consistent and effective global response to biohazard incidents. These standards cover various aspects of biohazard management, including safety procedures, remediation techniques, and environmental protection measures.

Key initiatives in the development of global standards and protocols include:

- **The International Health Regulations (IHR):** Revised in 2005, the IHR provides a legal framework for the international response to public health emergencies that have the potential to cross borders. The regulations emphasise the importance of reporting outbreaks, sharing information, and cooperating on public health measures.

- **ISO Standards for Biohazard Management:** The International Organisation for Standardisation (ISO) has developed several standards related to biohazard management, including ISO 35001 for bio risk management. These standards provide guidelines for the establishment and maintenance of bio risk management systems.

- **The Globally Harmonised System of Classification and Labelling of Chemicals (GHS):** The GHS is an international standard for the classification and labelling of chemicals, including hazardous chemicals that can pose biohazard risks. The GHS aims to ensure consistent communication of chemical hazards to promote safety in their handling, transport, and use.

The establishment of these and other international standards and protocols is a testament to the global community's commitment to enhancing biohazard remediation efforts. By adhering to these standards, countries and organisations can ensure that their biohazard management practices are aligned with the best available science and are effective in protecting public health and the environment.

Global perspectives and international cooperation are indispensable in the management of biohazard incidents. The interconnectedness of our world means that biohazards in one region can quickly become global crises. Through collaborative efforts, the sharing of resources and information, and adherence to international standards and protocols, the global community can enhance its resilience to biohazard threats. The case studies and initiatives discussed in this chapter highlight the progress that has been made in this area, as well as the ongoing need for cooperation and innovation in biohazard remediation.

## Asbestos Removal

Asbestos removal involves the safe and effective removal of asbestos containing materials from buildings and structures.

## Biohazard Cleaning

Biohazard cleaning is the process of cleaning, disinfecting and disposing of hazardous materials in a safe and appropriate manner.

## House Clearances

House clearances involve the removal and disposal of unwanted items and materials from residential properties.

## Commercial Cleaning

Commercial cleaning is a professional service that involves the cleaning and maintenance of commercial properties such as offices, shops, and warehouses.

## Legionella Remedial Works

Legionella treatment is the process of eliminating the bacteria responsible for Legionnaires' disease from water systems.

## Virus Decontamination

Virus decontamination involves the use of specialised techniques and equipment to remove viruses and other pathogens from surfaces reducing the risk of infection.

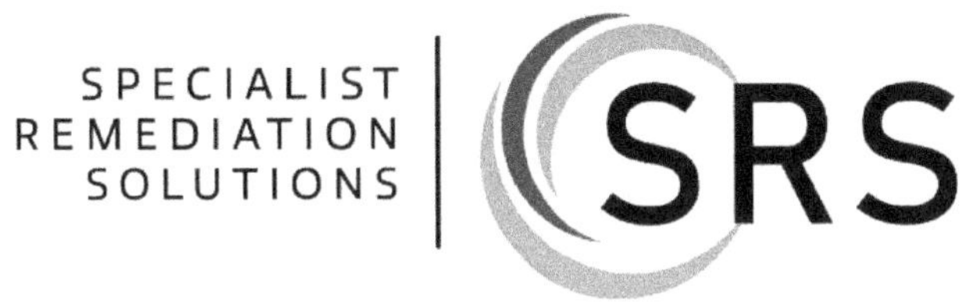


# DO YOU NEED HELP?

We provide asbestos removal, biohazard cleaning, house clearance, and commercial cleaning services, with a commitment to customer satisfaction through the use of the best equipment, materials, and techniques.

## GET IN CONTACT TODAY!

www.srsolutions.uk

T: 01536 860 166

E: info@srsolutionsltd.uk

# © 2024 COPYRIGHT STATEMENT